Copycat Recipes Making

Make Most Popular Sandwich at Home
(Famous Restaurant Copycat Cookbook)
Sandwich Maker Cookbook 2021

Your Essential Guide to Living the
Copycat Lifestyle

CECILIA LEWIS

Copyright © 2012 Cecilia Lewis

INTRODUCTION

Sandwiches are quick meals to prepare because they are nothing more than pieces of bread divided into two parts and which can be prepared with both simple and complex toppings.

now-days they are very popular in street food, where the sandwich has now become delicious and at the same time cheaper dish.

In this cookbook there are different types of sandwiches, slices of bread or even better bruschetta with recipes from all over the world and for all tastes, there are sandwiches for carnivores forceful spices and aromas, or there are sandwiches for pescatarian, with the best species of bluefish, or there are also sandwiches for vegans or vegetarians.

In short, inside you can indulge yourself with different types of sandwiches, which have now also become a simple dish not only for street food but a real way of life.

CONTENTS

CROUTONS IN SOUR-SWEET

for 4 people INGREDIENTS

- 8 slices of sandwich bread
- 100 g of raw ham
- 1 tablespoon of capers
- 1 tablespoon of pine nuts
- 1 tablespoon of raisins
- 1 teaspoon of sugar
- a little flour
- a little vinegar
- oil

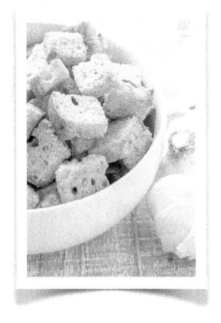

First you have to cut the bread into small rectangles. As soon as they are cut, they must be fried in hot oil and drained in absorbent paper. In a pan of flour, mix a tablespoon of sugar, then take the previously mixed content and pour into a bowl and toast the content over low heat.

In the meantime, add half a glass of water with vinegar, in the meantime it must always be stirred until it boils.

To complete it all you have to add capers, pine nuts, raisins and finally ham cut into small pieces.

At the end of the entire preparation and cooking process, distribute all the contents on the croutons and serve immediately.

BACON CROUTONS

for 2 people INGREDIENTS

- 6 crusty round bread rolls
- 6 slices of bacon
- 6 slices of cheese (like pickles)
- 10 g of butter
- mustard

PREPARATION

First, brown the slices of bread in the middle of the butter, when they are well browned, dry them with absorbent paper and distribute some mustard, while cutting slices of cheese of the same shape as the bread already cut previously and lay them on the crust. Meanwhile, grill the slices of bacon and spread it on the croutons. Finally, you have to heat everything in the oven and wait until the cheese melts with the croutons and serve immediately.

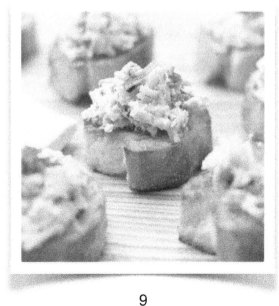

HOT CHICKEN CROUTONS

serves 6 INGREDIENTS

- 12 VERY THIN slices of cooked chicken breast

- 6 slices of bread

- 6 thinly sliced pickled cucumbers

- 12 tablespoons of grated Parmesan cheese

- butter, salt, pepper to taste

PREPARATION

Spread a layer of butter on the freshly toasted slices of bread, immediately after add two slices of chicken on the slices of bread and season with salt, pepper and oil as required.

In the meantime, add a few slices of cucumber on the bread and put a tablespoon of flaked Parmesan cheese and bake everything at 210° for about 10 minutes or until the cheese has melted and becomes golden. Now serve hot.

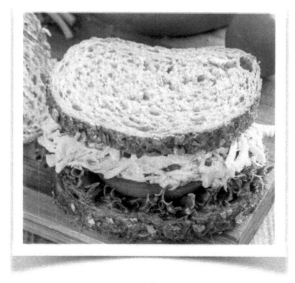

TURKEY CROUTONS

for 6 people INGREDIENTS

- 250 g of cooked turkey cut into squares

- 6 slices of bread (ALSO WHOLEMEAL)

- 100 g of chopped celery

- 70 g of mayonnaise

- butter

- 3 egg whites

- 50 g of grated Parmesan cheese

- salt, pepper to taste

- 1 and 1/2 tablespoons of lemon juice

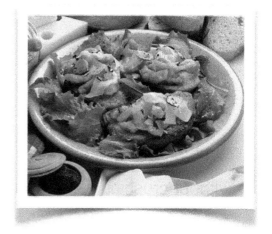

PREPARATION

Take a medium-sized pot and put some lemon juice, mayonnaise, celery and finally the turkey, over low heat add salt, pepper and oil as required. In the meantime that the turkey is cooking, we have to toast the slices of bread, but be careful, only on one side, instead on the other side, not toasted, we have to spread the turkey seasoning.

Whisk the egg whites, add a spoonful of Parmesan cheese and carefully pour the turkey mixture, mixing it slowly.

Toast the croutons in the oven at 200° for about 10 minutes until golden and puffy.

HAMBURGERS

for 4 people INGREDIENTS

- 4 soft round rolls

- 550 g of lean ground beef

- 1 tablespoon of oil - salt, pepper

PREPARATION

Put the meat in a bowl and season with pepper and salt as required, but without crushing it very much. Prepare the dough of the same shape in 4 or more very thick medallions, grilled by adding a drizzle of oil, leaving them a little pink inside.

The hamburger must be served inside the sandwiches and can be seasoned according to your taste, with mustard, raw onion, salad etc.

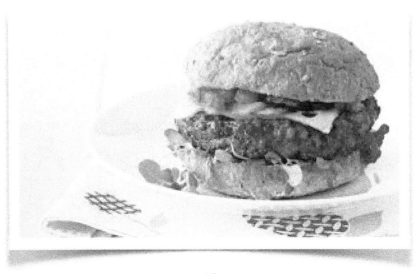

HOT DOG

for 4 people INGREDIENTS

- 8 small oval rolls

- 4 frankfurters

- 8 slices of smoked bacon

- 4 pickled gherkins

PREPARATION

The sausage and cucumbers must be cut in half. Meanwhile wrap the sausage and half cucumber with a slice of bacon and cook at 200° for about 12 minutes or until the bacon is browned. Finally cut the sandwiches in half and put the sausage with the freshly baked bacon. Serve immediately.

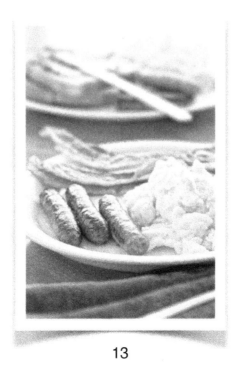

COOKED HAM SANDWICH

for 4 people INGREDIENTS

- 8 slices of bread like Merano

- 4 slices of 100 g of cooked ham

- 4 cucumbers cut into slices

- 50 g of butter

- Tabasco

PREPARATION

Mix some butter with a few drops of Tabasco (just enough) spread it on each slice of bread, then place a few slices of ham and cucumber, finally cover with another slice of bread and serve.

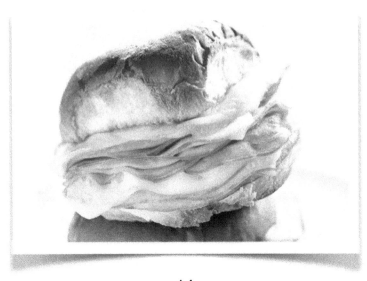

VEAL AND HAM BUNS

for 4 people INGREDIENTS

- 4 loaf-shaped sandwiches

- 4 slices of roast veal of about 80 g each

- 100 g of raw ham cut into wide strips

- 40 g of butter

- Worcestershire sauce

PREPARATION

Remove the breadcrumbs after cutting them in two parts, then mix the Worcestershire sauce with the butter to obtain a creamy mixture. Spread the mixture on the slice of bread and put a slice of ham and a slice of roast. Serve.

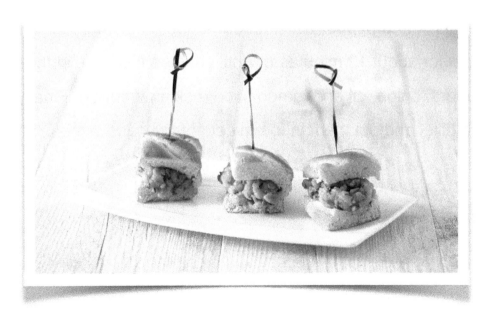

TARTARE SANDWICH

serves 4 INGREDIENTS

- 8 milk sandwiches

- 320 g of beef fillet

- 1/2 lemon

- 1 small onion

- 1 teaspoon of mustard

- 1 splash of Worcestershire sauce

- 1 tablespoon of capers - butter

- oil, salt, pepper

PREPARATION

Cut the sandwiches in half by carefully removing the crumb inside them, immediately afterwards butter and season with Worcestershire sauce, mustard, salt and pepper as required. In the meantime, cook the fillet at 200° and for about 12 minutes or until you see it brown, in the meantime add capers, onion, oil and lemon juice making it soften. Finally, take the slices of fillet and put them in the middle of the sandwiches. Serve.

ROASTED SANDWICH

for 4 people INGREDIENTS

- 4 sandwiches

- 4 slices of roast veal or beef

- 2 anchovy fillets

- 1 tablespoon of chopped parsley

- 1 knob of butter

PREPARATION

Put the anchovies, parsley and butter in a medium-sized bowl, mix everything well. Meanwhile, cook the roast until they brown it. Cut the sandwiches in half and spread the mixture on each individual sandwich. As soon as the roast is ready, place it in the middle of the sandwiches and serve immediately.

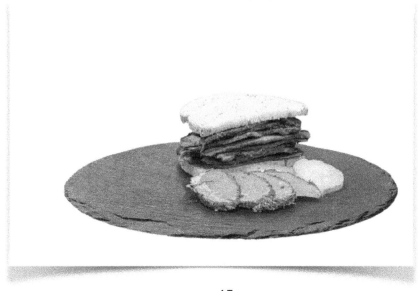

SANDWICH WITH ROAST TOMATO AND CUCUMBERS

for 4 people INGREDIENTS

- 8 slices of bread

- 100 g of sliced roast veal

- 3 tablespoons of mayonnaise

- 1 large tomato

- 1 fresh cucumber

- salt, pepper

PREPARATION

Cut a cucumber into slices and sprinkle it with salt, let it rest for about 50 minutes so that its water drips, as soon as the salting time has elapsed, rinse it with cold water and dry it. Immediately after spreading the mayonnaise on the sandwich and put slices of tomato and cucumber, finally add the slices of roast previously cooked in a pan with very little oil. Serve immediately.

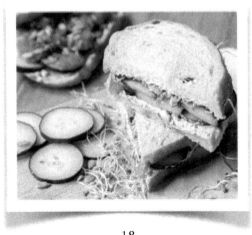

SANDWICH WHIT CANNED MEAT

for 4 people INGREDIENTS

- 4 sandwiches1 box of meat

- 4 lettuce leaves

- 4 pickled cucumbers

- 2 tablespoons of capers

- 2 tablespoons of mayonnaise

PREPARATION

Cut the sandwiches in half and spread mayonnaise on them. Meanwhile, cook the meat in a pan, adding very little oil. When ready, take the sandwiches and add a spoonful of capers, the sliced cucumber, and a lettuce leaf. When ready, serve immediately.

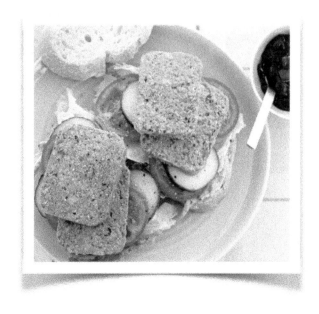

SANDWICH WHIT HAM AND PINEAPPLE

for 4 people INGREDIENTS

- 4 sandwiches

- 4 thick slices of cooked ham

- 4 slices of pineapple

- butter

PREPARATION

After cutting the sandwiches in half, butter them in one part only. Put the pineapple slices with the cooked ham in the middle of the sandwich, close it with the other half and put it in the oven for just a few minutes, to serve hot.

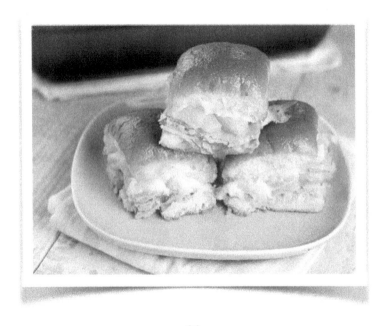

SANDWICH WHIT HAM AND MUSTARD

for 4 people INGREDIENTS

- 200 g of butter

- 2 tablespoons of mustard

- 4 slices of cooked ham

- finely grated onions

- 4 sandwiches

PREPARATION

Mix the butter with the mustard in a small pan until we obtain a homogeneous cream. Open the sandwiches in half and spread with the buttercream, add the grated onion, and the cooked ham. Serve.

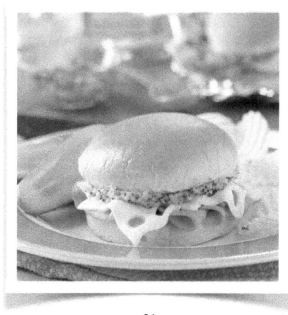

SANDWICH WHIT ROAST BEEF AND LETTUCE

for 4 people INGREDIENTS

- 8 slices of Tuscan bread

- 4 slices of roast beef of 80 g each

- 4 fresh lettuce leaves

- 40 g of butter

- 1 teaspoon of mustard

- coarse ground black pepper

PREPARATION

Work the butter with the mustard in a pan until it becomes a creamy mixture. Meanwhile, cook the roast beef in a pan to make it crisp and add a little black pepper. As soon as the roast beef is cooked, spread the mixture on the slices of bread and place the meat inside the sandwich and add a lettuce leaf. Serve still hot.

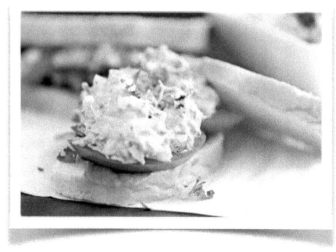

ARTIST SANDWICH

for 4 people INGREDIENTS

- 8 slices of sandwich bread

- 50 g of butter

- 150 g of cooked ham

- 50 g of cured tongue

- 2 hard-boiled eggs

PREPARATION

Toast the slices of bread in the oven. In the meantime, chop the hard-boiled eggs with the tongue and ham. As soon as the slices of bread are toasted, spread the butter and add the chopped mixture. Serve on a plate and serve.

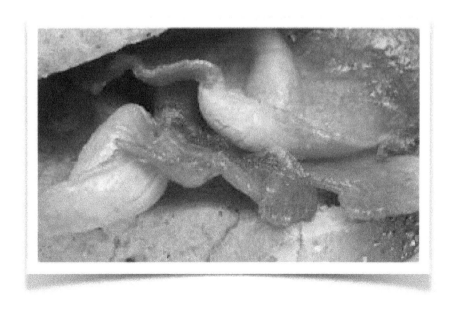

PORK ARIST SANDWICH

for 4 people INGREDIENTS

- 8 slices of Tuscan bread

- 4 slices of roasted pork loin of 80 g each

- 50 g of butter

- 1 tablespoon of mustard

- 8 tomato slices

- 4 sliced pickled gherkins

- lettuce leaves

PREPARATION

To get a homogeneous cream, mix the butter with the mustard and spread it on the four slices of bread. In the meantime, cook the loin in a pan to do first, until golden brown, immediately afterward place a lettuce leaf on the slices of bread and then the freshly cooked loin. Finally, season with tomato and cucumber slices, cover with another slice of bread, and serve.

CHICKEN SANDWICH

for 4 people INGREDIENTS

- 8 slices of sandwich bread

- 300 g of boiled chicken breast

- 1 tablespoon of butter

- 1 teaspoon of mustard

- thin slices of tomato

- salt

PREPARATION

Take the previously boiled chicken breast and clean it from any bones or cartilage, then cut it into thin slices. Mix the butter with the mustard. Remove the crust from the bread and spread and spread the slices of bread with the buttercream.

Take the chicken and spread it on half of the slices of bread and on the thin slices of tomato previously sprinkled with salt to make them lose their water. Cover with the other slices, press them lightly, and serve.

SANDWICH FOIE GRAS

for 4 people INGREDIENTS

- 1 sliced 1/2 kg sliced bread

- 100 g butter

- 1 tablespoon of anchovy paste

- 200 g of black olives

- 200 g of foie gras pate

PREPARATION

Remove the bread crust and cut two triangles from each slice. Mix the butter with the anchovy paste until you get a thick cream. Spread a third of the bread with the pate and cream of anchovies and butter and chopped olives on the remaining triangles. Take the triangles with the olives and overlap each one with a triangle with the butter and anchovy cream and one with the pate. Finally, insert each sandwich with a toothpick and serve.

SANDWICH WHIT SAUSAGE

for 4 people INGREDIENTS

- 8 thin slices of rye bread

- 12 thin slices of sausage

- 3 tablespoons of butter

- 1 tablespoon of horseradish sauce

- thin slices of radish

PREPARATION

Mix the butter with the horseradish sauce until creamy and light, then spread it on the four slices of rye bread. Stuff the slices of bread with radishes and sausage, then reassemble with the other slices of bread. To serve.

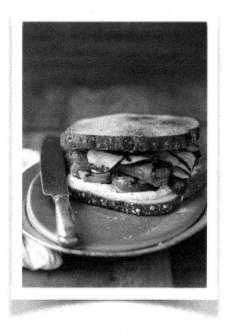

AMERICAN SANDWICH

for 4 people INGREDIENTS

- slices of bread and 150 g. of butter
- slices of salted tongue
- 20 scampi - 2 firm tomatoes
- 1 head of lettuce
- 4 eggs 1 lemon Worcestershire sauce
- mayonnaise, oil salt, pepper

PREPARATION

Mix the butter with salt, pepper, and two drops of Worcestershire sauce until you get a thick cream. Add the previously cooked and sifted prawns, then mix well. Spread the cream on the slices of bread, remove the crust from the bread and toast them lightly. Boil 3 eggs. Beat a raw egg yolk with salt and pepper and mix it with lemon juice and 1 dl of oil. Grease the slices of bread, put 3 slices of tomato and a few lettuce leaves on top, immediately after spreading the mayonnaise on each slice of bread, butter and toast the other slice. Put a slice of tongue on these. Now arrange the slices of hard-boiled eggs and garnish with the prawns and a little mayonnaise. Close the sandwiches with the last slices of toast with the buttered side inwards. Secure with toothpicks and serve.

CHICKEN AND WATERCRESS PATE' SANDWICH

for 4 people INGREDIENTS

- watercress mayonnaise to taste

- 200 g of chicken breast cooked and thinly sliced for the curry butter:

- 125 g of butter

- 2 tablespoons of curry powder

- salt

PREPARATION

Freeze the bread in the freezer for 2 hours, remove the crust and cut it on the long side into slices about 0.5 cm thick. In a bowl, mix the soft butter with the curry and a pinch of salt, spread the side of the longer slices with this mixture.

Put the sprigs of watercress that you have washed and dried and spread with the mayonnaise. Spread the chicken slices with a little mayonnaise. Add some more watercress and cover with the remaining slices of bread with the buttered side underneath. Arrange the slices on top of each other, cover with a damp cloth, and keep them in the refrigerator to cool. Cut the slices short to form sticks about 3/4 cm wide, arrange them on a serving dish and serve.

AMERICAN SANDWICH 2

for 4 people INGREDIENTS

- slices of bread 150 grams of butter

- slices of corned tongue

- 20 shrimp fish

- 2 firm tomatoes

- 1 head of lettuce

- 4 eggs - 1 lemon

- Worcestershire sauce

- mayonnaise to taste

- oil, salt, pepper

PREPARATION

Mix the butter into a cream and season with salt, pepper, and two drops of Worcestershire sauce. Add the previously cooked prawns and mix well. Spread the mixture on the slices of bread, remove the crust and lightly toast them.

Boil 3 eggs. Beat a raw egg yolk with salt and pepper and mix it with lemon juice and 1 dl of oil.

Grease four slices of bread, place 1 lettuce leaf and 3 tomato slices on top, then spread the mayonnaise on top and place on each other slice of buttered and toasted bread.

Place a slice of tongue on the slices of bread, then the hard-boiled eggs and garnish with the prawns and a little mayonnaise. Close the sandwiches with the slices of toast with the buttered side inwards and serve.

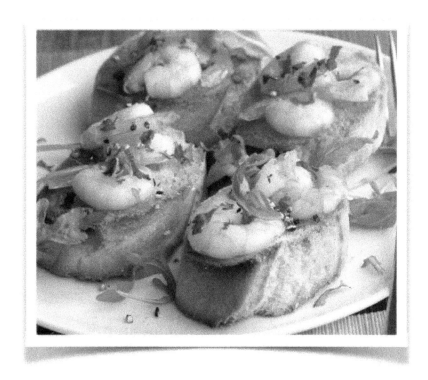

SANDWICH WHIT CHICKEN PATE AND WATERCRESS

for 4 people INGREDIENTS

- fresh bread

- bunches of watercress

- mayonnaise to taste

- 200 g of chicken breast cooked and thinly sliced for the curry butter:

- 125 g of butter

- 2 tablespoons of curry powder - salt

PREPARATION

Put the whole bread in the freezer for 2 hours, then remove the crust and cut it lengthwise into slices about 0.6 cm thick. Then you have to mix the curry with butter and a pinch of salt, then spread one side of the long slices with the cream got. Take the slices of bread and spread the mayonnaise and put the sprigs of watercress, but after having washed and dried them. Take the chicken slices and spread the mayonnaise on them and put them on the slice of bread, then add a little more watercress and cover with the remaining slices of bread with the buttered side. Close the slices of bread and place them on a damp cloth and put them in the refrigerator to cool them. Finally, cut the bread to get several slices and serve on a serving dish.

SANDWICH WHIT CURRY LAMB

for 4 people INGREDIENTS

- 4 thick slices of wholemeal bread
- 300 g of diced baby lamb or cooked lamb
- 1 small onion, finely chopped
- 2 tablespoons of butter
- 1 tablespoon of flour
- 1 tablespoon of curry powder
- 1/8 liter of chicken broth
- 50 ml of thick white yogurt
- 60 g of coarsely chopped toasted almonds
- salt, pepper - long strips of cucumber for garnish

PREPARATION

Fry the onion in butter, add the flour, the curry powder and cook, stirring constantly, for about 1 minute. While simmering for 5 minutes, you need to add the chicken broth and keep stirring. Then add the lamb, yogurt and season with salt and pepper; heat without bringing it to a boil. Take the slices of bread and toast them on one side only, then spread the untoasted side with butter and divide the cream got with the lamb on top. Put on a serving dish and garnish with cucumber and serve.

SANDWICH WHIT CHICKEN LIVER AND APPLES

for 4 people INGREDIENTS

- 1/2 kg of clean chicken livers

- 8 slices of wholemeal bread

- 1 thinly sliced onion

- 1 golden apple - 60 ml of Tawny port

- 6 tablespoons of butter - salt, pepper - slices of boiled egg

PREPARATION

Take a pan and put the livers in the butter and cook for 3-4 minutes to obtain the browning on the outside and season with salt and pepper. As soon as the livers turn golden, remove them from the pan and put the peeled and chopped apple with onion, and cook for about ten minutes, stirring occasionally. Add the livers again and bring to the boil until the mixture is thicker and creamy. In the end, let the puree cool in the blender and correct with salt and pepper. Leave to cool in the refrigerator to get a more concentrated cream. Before serving the sandwiches, spread the slices of bread on them, lay thin slices of hard-boiled egg on them, and put the sandwiches back together with the other slices. To serve.

SANDWICH WHIT POLENTA

for 4 people INGREDIENTS

- 1 roll of pre-cooked polenta

- 8 thick slices of salami

- 8 pitted olives

- butter

PREPARATION

Slice the polenta to get 16 slices, then butter them on one side. Place one of the salami slices on half of the slices; cover the salami with a slice of polenta. Take the sandwiches got and fix them with toothpicks and an olive to decorate them. To serve.

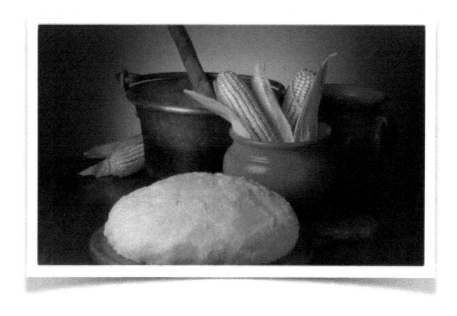

SANDWICH WHIT HAM AND SAUCE WHIT PEPPERS

for 4 people INGREDIENTS

- 4 slices of rye bread - butter

- 200 g of thinly sliced cooked ham

- 4 large lettuce leaves for the sauce

- 75 g of grated pecorino cheese

- 50 g of finely chopped pickled red pepper - 1/2 cup of milk - 1 - tablespoon of flour - 1 tablespoon of butter - salt, Cayenne pepper

PREPARATION

Melt the butter in a pan, add the flour and cook for 3 minutes, stirring constantly. As soon as three minutes have passed, remove them from the heat and add some milk and mix until you get a creamy and homogeneous mixture, add salt and pepper. Let the sauce cook for 5 minutes, adding the cheese a little at a time and stirring to let it melt. Add the cayenne pepper and more salt and pepper to taste.

Spread the slices of bread with a layer of butter; put the lettuce and ham on top. Finally, cover the slices of bread with other slices and arrange the sandwiches on a serving plate, heat the plate, and sprinkle it with the sauce. Serve immediately.

SANDWICH WHIT ROAST

for 4 people INGREDIENTS

- 8 slices of homemade bread

- 8 slices of cold roast veal

- 4 tablespoons of remoulade sauce

- 4 lettuce leaves

- 8 thin slices of tomato butter, salt

PREPARATION

Butter the slices after removing the bread crust. After washing the lettuce, dry it and place it on the bread. Then put a slice of roast on the lettuce and spread the meat with the sauce. Cut the tomato into thin slices, add salt to taste and cover everything with the other slice of bread, press it and serve.

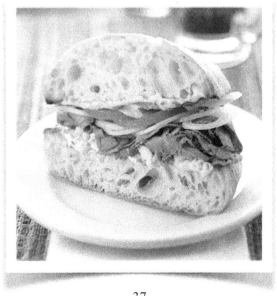

FANCY SANDWICH

for 4 people INGREDIENTS

- 16 slices of sandwich bread

- 100 g of cooked ham

- 200 g of mayonnaise

- 2 tomatoes

- 1 small lettuce

- 2 eggs - 2 tablespoons of olive paté - butter - salt

PREPARATION

Prepare an omelet with 2 eggs, a little butter, and a pinch of salt. Melt the olive pate with the butter and try to obtain a homogeneous cream. Spread a layer of butter on only one of the four slices of bread.

Add a slice of ham on top; cover them with another slice of ham cut in the same shape as the slice of bread. Put the other slice of bread on top and spread the paté previously worked with butter on top and cover with half an omelet. On this place the third slice of bread and spread it with a little mayonnaise by adding a lettuce leaf and a few thin slices of tomato on top. Season the other sandwiches in the same way.

TASTY SANDWICH

for 4 people INGREDIENTS

- 8 slices of sandwich bread

- 1 cacciatorino

- 16 small frankfurters

- 16 pitted olives

- butter a few leaves of salad

PREPARATION

Cut the eight slices of bread in half to get sixteen equal triangles, greasing them with butter and placing a salad leaf on each one making sure it is the same size as the triangle. Then cut the cacciatorino (salami). Take the sausage and put it on top of the salami slices, finally fix everything with a toothpick and an olive as decoration.

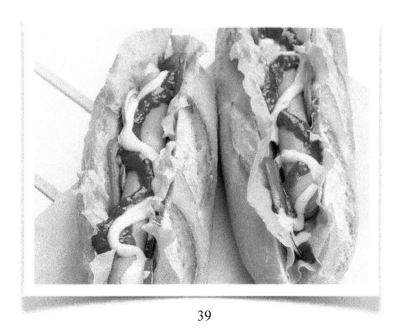

TASTY CHEESE SANDWICH

for 4 people INGREDIENTS

- 4 soft round rolls

- 500 g of lean ground beef

- 4 thin slices of cheese

- oil, salt and pepper

PREPARATION

Combine the meat with salt, pepper and mix well, get from the dog four medallions of the same shape as the sandwiches and very thick. Meanwhile, toast the sandwiches on one side only. Cook the meat in a pan on one side only and place it in the already toasted sandwiches. Cover with a slice of cheese and cook until the cheese has melted. Add mustard, lettuce, ketchup, chili sauce, and onion to your liking. To serve.

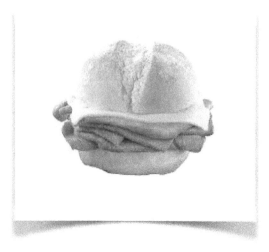

CROUTONS GRUYERE

for 4 people INGREDIENTS

- 4 slices of freshly stale sandwich bread

- 4 slices of gruyere

- 4 slices of cooked ham

- 4 tablespoons of thick béchamel

- 1 egg yolk

- butter

PREPARATION

Take the slices of bread and toast them with butter in a pan. Remove the bread crust from the slices and add the ham cut in the same shape as the slices of bread. Spread with the béchamel and add the egg yolk, then cover with the slices of Gruyere and put them to heat to melt the cheese slightly. This sandwich could be seasoned to your liking with different variations.

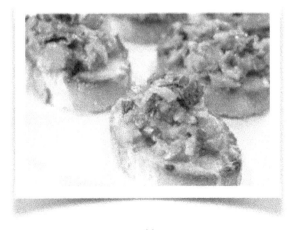

CHEESE CROUTONS WHIT TRUFFLES

for 4 people INGREDIENTS

- 8 slices of sandwich bread

- 100 g of Bel Paese cut into thin slices

- 50 g of butter

- 1 truffle

PREPARATION

Take the bread and get triangular slices. Put the butter in a bowl and add the truffle, work it with a wooden spoon to get a soft cream. Cut the cheese into the same shape as the slices of bread. Finally, take the croutons and spread with the truffle butter and distribute sliced cheese. Serve as an appetizer.

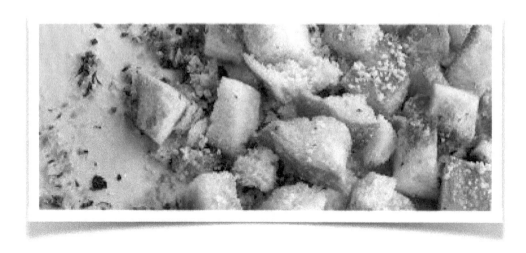

CROUTONS WHIT MOZZARELLA

for 6 people INGREDIENTS

- 24 slices of stale bread

- 12 slices of buffalo mozzarella

- 3 eggs

- 5 tablespoons of milk - flour, oil, salt

PREPARATION

Take the mozzarella and cut it to the same size as the croutons and place the mozzarella in the middle of the slices of bread.

Flour the croutons and place them in a bowl with beaten egg, milk and salt, leave enough for them to absorb the mixture.

Finally fry them in a pan with oil and serve hot.

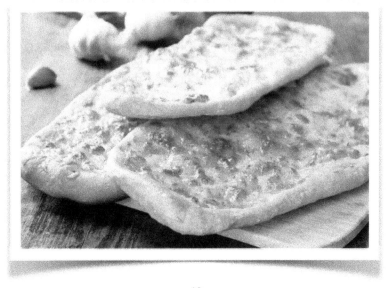

CAMEMBERT SANDWICH

for 4 people INGREDIENTS

- 4 sandwiches

- 150 g of camembert

- 100 g of butter

- 1 banana

- the juice of 1/2 lemon to decorate

- 20 toasted almond fillets

- 16 mustard cherries

- 16 mandarin wedges

PREPARATION

Take the Camembert and pass it through the food processor, add the butter a little at a time until you get a homogeneous cream. Meanwhile toast the sandwiches and spread the cream cheese and butter.

Cut a banana into slices and sprinkle it with lemon juice, then place it on the rolls, pressing them lightly. Finally decorated with mandarin, cherries and almonds and serve.

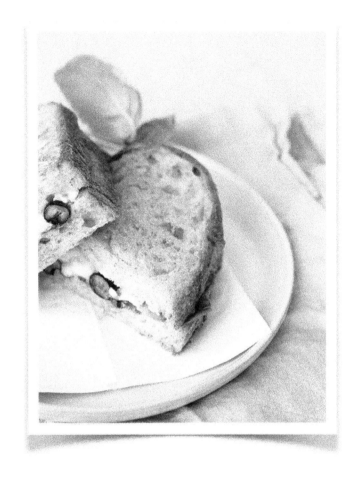

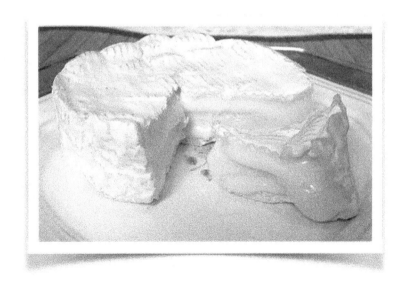

MOZZARELLA IN A CARRIAGE

for 6 people INGREDIENTS

- 12 slices of cow's milk

- 24 slices of bread

- 3 eggs

- 1/2 glass of milk - flour breadcrumbs - oil, salt

PREPARATION

Cut the mozzarella and dry it slightly, then cut it to the same size as the bread and place it in the middle of the slices.

Take a small pan and beat the eggs with the milk and a pinch of salt, then dip the sandwich and sprinkle it with flour, until they become softer.

Then press them well and pass them once again in the breadcrumbs, then fry in a pan with hot oil and serve.

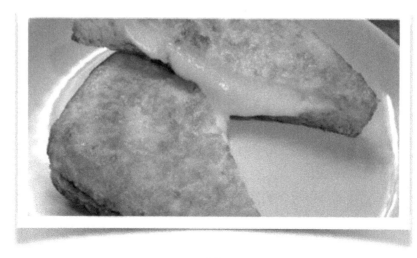

MOZZARELLA IN CARRIAGE 2

for 6 people INGREDIENTS

- 24 slices of stale bread

- 12 slices of buffalo mozzarella

- 3 eggs

- 5 tablespoons of milk - flour, oil, salt

PREPARATION

This recipe has the same procedure as the previous one, only the mozzarella changes. You just have to be careful to dry the buffalo mozzarella because it has a lot of liquid milk. Cut the mozzarella and dry it slightly, then cut it to the same size as the bread and place it in the middle of the slices. Take a small pan and beat the eggs with the milk and a pinch of salt, then dip the sandwich and sprinkle it with flour, until they become softer. Then press them well and pass them once again in the breadcrumbs, then fry in a pan with hot oil and serve.

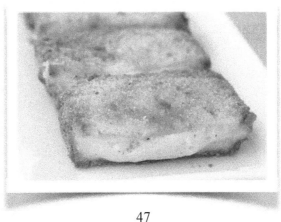

COMINO SANDWICH

for 4 people INGREDIENTS

- 8 slices of sandwich bread

- 8 slices of emmental

- 50 g of butter1 pinch of paprika

- 1 teaspoon of cumin

- seeds dry white wine

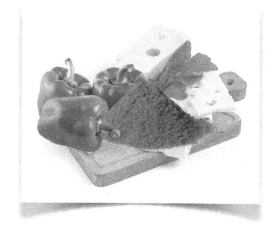

PREPARATION

Take the sandwiches and remove the rib of bread, butter it on one side and wet it with white wine (use what you have at home).

Place a slice of Emmental on each half of the bun, then place the slices of bread on a greased baking sheet and heat slowly until the cheese has melted

Eliminate the bread crust; spread it on one side with melted butter and on the other wet it with white wine. Place a slice of Emmental on each.

Finally, serve with a pinch of paprika and sprinkle with cumin seeds.

CHEESE AND SALAMI SANDWICH

for 4 people INGREDIENTS

- 8 slices of bread

- 4 slices of fontina

- 100 g of sliced salami

- 50 g of butter

PREPARATION

Peel the salami and remove the crust from the bread immediately after spread the slices of bread with butter and put a slice of cheese on it and then the salami to taste. Finally cover everything with the other slice of sandwich and serve.

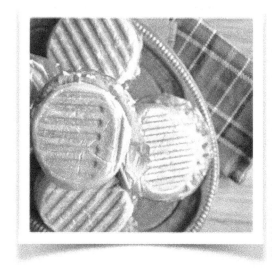
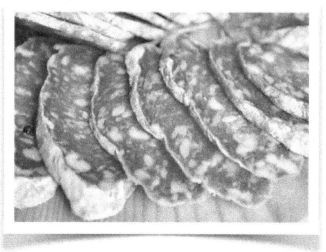

GORGONZOLA SANDWICH

for 4 people INGREDIENTS

- 8 slices of bread

- 120 g of sweet gorgonzola

- 60 g of butter

- 1 tablespoon of chopped parsley

PREPARATION

Work the gorgonzola (cheese) by pouring it into a bowl with the butter and mix it with a spatula to get a creamy mixture. When the mixture is ready, add some chopped parsley and mix well.

Finally, take the freshly prepared mixture once again and spread it on the slices of bread, then cover it with the remaining slices and serve.

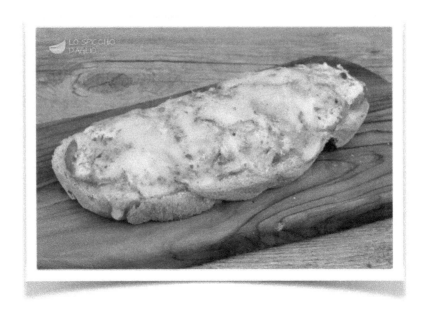

ROQUEFORT SANDWICH

for 4 people INGREDIENTS

- 4 slices of wholemeal or rye bread

- 60 g of Roquefort cheese

- 100 g of soft white Philadelphia cheese

- butter

PREPARATION

Mix the white cheese with the Roquefort to get a homogeneous mixture. In the meantime, take the bread and toast it on the grill until it is lightly browned. As soon as the bread is ready, spread the mixture got previously and spread a light layer of butter, and put them back on the grill for two minutes at the most to get a good browning. Finally, cut it into several parts and distribute hot.

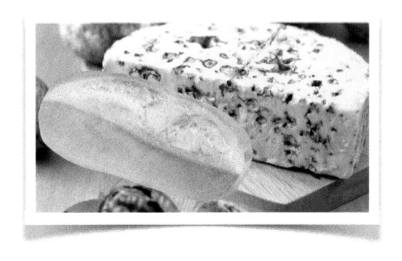

SANDWICH TALEGGIO AND LARD

for 4 people INGREDIENTS

- 100 g of taleggio cheese

- 100 g of smoked lard

- a pinch of paprika

- 1 tablespoon of capers

- 8 slices of rye bread

PREPARATION

Take a meat grinder and put the taleggio, the lard with the paprika and finally the capers, work the mixture until it becomes creamy. Meanwhile, take the bread and toast it.

As soon as you have finished chopping everything, put the mixture on the slices of bread and cover them with the other slices. Serve hot.

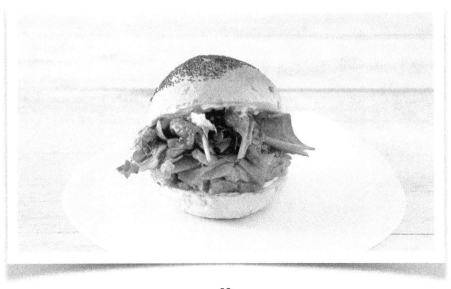

CREAM SANDWICH

for 4 people INGREDIENTS

- 4 finger-high slices of bread

- butter

- 1 of cream

- 1 tablespoon of grated Parmesan cheese

- 4 slices of gruyere

PREPARATION

Take the rolls and remove the crust, then butter them with a little butter on both sides. Put them on the pan and wait for them to turn golden. Meanwhile, add the Parmesan cheese with the whipped cream and mix gently until you get a thick cream. As soon as the slices of bread are golden brown, spread the cream previously got and place the thin slices of Gruyere on top. Serve on a serving plate.

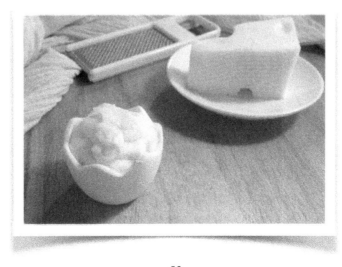

GROVIERA (CHEESE) SANDWICH

for 4 people INGREDIENTS

- 8 soft rolls

- 1/2 glass of milk

- 150 g of grated Gruyere cheese

- 1 egg yolk

- 3 slices of cooked ham

PREPARATION

Take the sandwiches and cut them in half, now remove the excess crumb with a spoon. Then take the breadcrumbs and put it in a bowl with hot milk and add an egg yolk and a little grated Gruyere cheese.

Finally, cut the ham into small pieces, add it together with the breadcrumbs and milk, then mix everything. Immediately after, stuff the sandwiches and serve them with or without the cap.

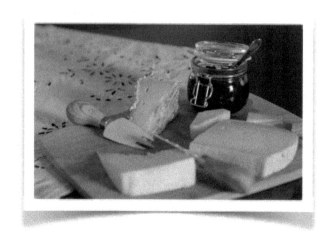

SWISS SANDWICH

for 4 people INGREDIENTS

- 8 slices of sandwich bread

- 8 slices of gruyere

- 1 onion

- 50 g of butter

- mustard

- paprika

- little oil

PREPARATION

Put the butter in a pan and fry it with the addition of paprika and oil as required.

In the meantime, toast the bread and wait for it to become slightly golden, as soon as it is ready, place the onion and gruyere on each slice, bake to let the cheese melt. Serve immediately, adding mustard to taste.

STRACCHINO (CHEESE) SANDWICH

for 4 people INGREDIENTS

- 8 slices of bread

- 130 g of stracchino

- 60 g of butter

- a few chopped walnut kernels

- a pinch of powdered mixed spices - salt

PREPARATION

Mix the stracchino in a bowl and add the butter, trying to get a thick and homogeneous cream.Season the mixture with a pinch of salt and spices and add the walnuts.Finally, distribute the cream got on the slices of bread and cover them with the top of the sandwiches and serve..

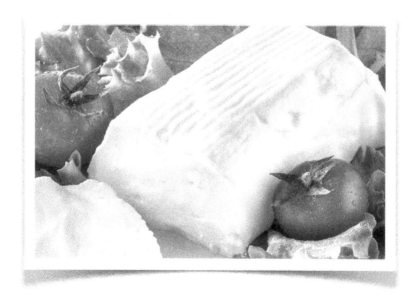

SANDWICH (CHEESE) WHIT FONTINA AND PEPPER

for 4 people INGREDIENTS

- 8 slices of bread

- 100 g of fontina cheese cut into strips

- 1/2 fresh red pepper

- 40 g of butter

- salt, pepper

PREPARATION

Cut the pepper into strips and toast it in the oven. Then take a bowl and put some butter with salt and pepper in it. As soon as you have got a homogeneous mixture, spread it on the slices of bread and a few slices of fontina cheese cut into thin slices, season with fresh paprika and cover with the other slices of bread. To serve.

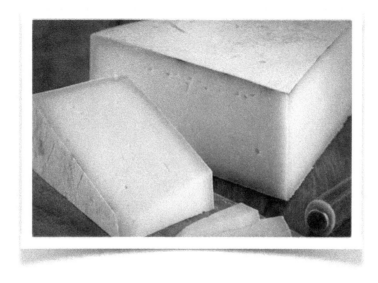

SANDWICH WHIT RICOTTA AND SPINACH

for 4 people INGREDIENTS

- 4 sandwiches

- 120 g of spinach

- 2 tablespoons of oil

- 1 piece of spring onion

- 250 g of ricotta - milk, salt, pepper, tomato

PREPARATION

Wash the spinach well and cook them in a pan with oil and salt for about five minutes. As soon as they have cooled, add a spring onion, salt, pepper and ricotta. Chop everything until you get a thick pulp and add the milk to moisten the pan. Crush the mixture to remove excess broth and fill the sandwiches. Then serve them on a serving dish..

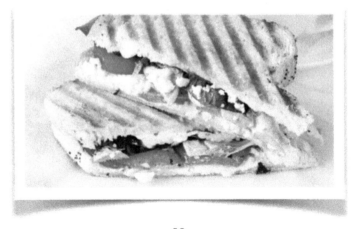

SANDWICH WHIT MOZZARELLA AND CAPERS

for 4 people INGREDIENTS

- 4 sandwiches

- 1 large mozzarella

- 3 tablespoons of oil

- chopped parsley

- 2 anchovy fillets, chopped

- 1/2 tablespoon of chopped capers

- 1 tablespoon of grated Parmesan cheese

- oregano

PREPARATION

Take the mozzarella and cut it into slices, then arrange it on a single plane. Then take a bowl and add the capers, oil, salt, parsley, oregano and anchovies, mixing everything trying to get a creamy mixture. Just finished, spread the mixture on the mozzarella.

Then take the sandwiches and remove the crumb, then lay the mozzarella on the slices of bread and keep in the fridge for about thirty minutes before serving.

ROQUEFORT SANDWICH AND TOMATO

for 4 people INGREDIENTS

- 1 aubergine of 400 g

- 120 g of crushed bread

- 200 g of Roquefort or other blue-veined cheese

- 4 slices of dark bread

- 3 tablespoons of butter plus spread

- 4 large, thick slices of tomato

- chopped fresh chives

PREPARATION

Before removing the tomatoes from the saucepan, sprinkle them with the grated cheese and wait for it to melt.

Finally, take the tomato and arrange it on the slices of bread, then lightly impregnate it with the cooking sauce and add the chopped chives.

Before serving, place it on a serving dish.

CHEESE AND EGGPLANT SANDWICH

for 4 people INGREDIENTS

- 100 g of grated scamorza cheese

- 50 g of finely chopped cooked ham

- 2 tablespoons of grated Parmesan cheese

- 1 egg and 2 egg yolks

- oil, flour breadcrumbs - chopped basil - salt, pepper

PREPARATION

Take the eggplant and peel it immediately after cutting it into eight slices, sprinkle it with salt and let it rest for about thirty minutes. Take a bowl and add the breadcrumbs, parmesan, ham, scamorza cheese, egg yolks, basil, salt and pepper to taste and mix everything together. Take a pan and brown the aubergines with a drizzle of oil as soon as they are ready, drain them with absorbent paper. At this point distribute the mixture with the cheese on the slices of bread and place the aubergines on top, then close them with the other slices of bread. Finally, after letting them cool in the fridge for at least half an hour, take a pan, pour a drizzle of oil and brown them slightly. Serve hot.

WHITE CHEESE AND OLIVE SANDWICH

for 6 people INGREDIENTS

- 4 sandwiches

- 8 very thin slices of wholemeal bread

- 4 very thin slices of white bread in very fresh boxes

- 4 very thin slices of rye bread

- 180 g of soft white Philadelphia cheese

- 80 g of pitted and chopped sweet black olives

- 3 spoons of butter

- 80 g of green olives stuffed with chopped pepper

- 80 g of chopped red pepper in oil

- 1 hard-boiled egg yolk

PREPARATION

Take a pan and mix two tablespoons of cheese, black olives, and a tablespoon of butter, use a food processor to get a nice creamy puree. In another bowl, place the green olives with the cheese and butter, always trying to get a homogeneous puree. Finally, put a pepper in another bowl, add two tablespoons of cheese, butter, and a hard-boiled egg. We now have three compounds. Now take the sandwiches and divide them in half, take the remaining cheese and sprinkle them with the black olive mixture, then cover it with a slice of white bread and spread the pepper mixture and cover it with a slice of rye and spread the green olive paste at the end cover with a slice of wholemeal bread and wrap it in plastic wrap. Prepare the rest of the sandwiches the same way and put them in the fridge for about an hour. Before serving, you can also remove the bread crust and cut the panini into triangles..

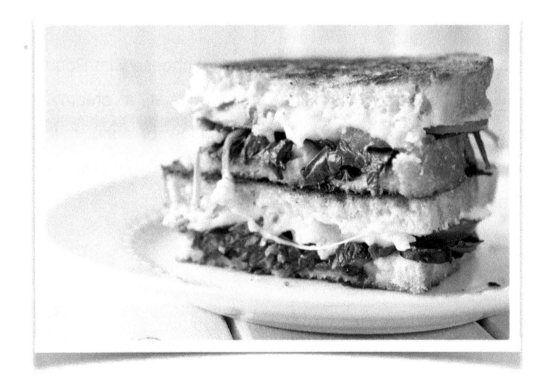

ROQUEFORT MOUSSE SANDWICH

for 4 people INGREDIENTS

- 4 sandwiches

- 1 fresh goat cheese

- 80 g of Roquefort

- 2 tablespoons of cognac

- 100 g of whipping cream

PREPARATION

Take a medium-sized pan and melt the goat cheese with Roquefort and a little cognac, mix everything until you get a creamy mixture. Meanwhile, keep the sandwiches in the fridge for about half an hour. Then whip the cream and try to add it gently, mixing slowly. At the end, stuff the sandwiches and serve them.

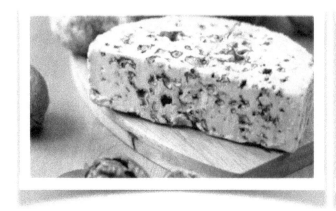
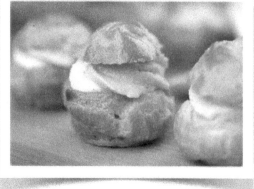

DUTCH CHEESE SANDWICH WITH APPLES

for 4 people INGREDIENTS

- 8 slices of sandwich bread

- 4 fairly thick slices of Gouda cheese

- 1 golden apple

- 4 tablespoons of butter

- 8 teaspoons of Dijon mustard

PREPARATION

Take the bread and remove its crust, then you need to cut the Gouda into the same shape as the bread.

Take an apple and cut it into slices, the same thickness of the cheese, then take a pan and put the butter, then brown the apple for about 5 minutes, now dry the apple with absorbent paper.

Take the bread and spread the mustard adding the apple and the slices of cheese, close the sandwiches and brown the bread in a pan with the butter until the cheese has melted. Finally mash them lightly with a spatula and cut the sandwiches into triangles. Serve.

ROQUEFORT AND NUTS SANDWICH

for 4 people INGREDIENTS

- 4 sandwiches

- 400 g of Roquefort cheese

- 100 g of white cream cheese like Philadelphia

- 2 tablespoons of cognac

- 60 g of finely chopped walnuts

- 8 slices of wholemeal bread

- butter sprigs of watercress

- small cherry tomatoes

PREPARATION

Melt the white cheese, Roquefort, Cognac and chopped walnuts in a bowl, mix well with a whisk until the mixture is homogeneous. Spread over the slices of bread and cover them with the remaining slices.

Finally, the two ends of the sandwiches must be spread with butter and browned in a pan.

Arrange the sandwiches on a serving dish and cut them in half to form equal triangles. at the end garnish the sandwiches with the sprigs of watercress and cherry tomatoes.

SUMMER SANDWICH

for 4 people INGREDIENTS

- 4 slices of bread

- 1 clove of garlic

- oil

- 400 g of ripe figs

- 6 anchovy fillets in oil

- 1 fresh onion

PREPARATION

First you have to toast the bread in the oven, immediately after sprinkle it with a drizzle of oil and rub the garlic on the slice. Now peel the figs and blend them with the anchovies, as soon as the mixture is ready, add a chopped onion. Finally, distribute the mixture got on the sandwiches and serve a serving dish.

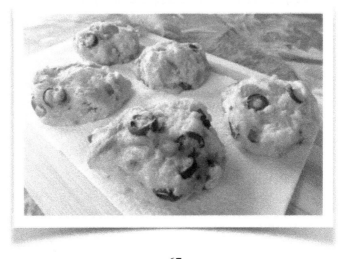

CROUTONS WITH SARDINES

for 8-9 people INGREDIENTS

- 150 g of sardines in olive oil

- 100 g of mayonnaise

- 2 teaspoons of lemon juice

- 20 g of finely chopped parsley

- Worcestershire sauce

- 18 fairly thick slices of French bread or loaf

- salt and pepper

PREPARATION

Dry the sardines and cut them into small pieces, then add the mayonnaise, Worcestershire sauce, lemon juice, salt and pepper to taste. Mix everything to get a consistent dough. Then spread all the dough on the slices of bread and bake at 200° for ten minutes or until the bread becomes crunchy. Then serve while hot.

HOT LOBSTER CROUTONS

for 6 people INGREDIENTS

- 230 g of cooked lobster pulp cut into small pieces

- 6 large slices of white bread for sandwiches

- 1/8 liter of béchamel sauce

- 1 and 1/2 teaspoons of tomato paste

- 1 teaspoon of lemon juice

- 1 tablespoon of grated gruyere - butter. salt and pepper

PREPARATION

Take a saucepan and thicken the béchamel, then take a bowl and put the tomato paste, the lemon juice and the béchamel itself, keep stirring until it becomes more homogeneous. Then add the lobster meat and season with salt and pepper. Now take the slices of bread and toast them on one side only. As soon as the bread is ready, try to create a disc of ten centimeters in diameter for each slice. Spread a light layer of butter on the side of the untoasted bread and add the lobster mixture, then sprinkle with the gruyere. Finally, place the croutons on the grill and cook them until the cheese melts.

CROUTONS CRAB AND TOMATO

for 6 people INGREDIENTS

- 150 g of well cleaned crab meat

- 6 slices of white bread

- 2 hard boiled eggs, chopped

- 50 g of mayonnaise - 6 thin slices of tomato

- 40 g of diced pickled cucumbers - 2 tablespoons of lemon juice

- 6 spoons of grated Parmesan cheese

- butter, Cayenne pepper, salt, white pepper

PREPARATION

Take a bowl and add the mayonnaise, egg, cucumber, crabmeat, lemon juice, cayenne pepper, salt and pepper to taste and mix everything until you get a creamy mixture. Meanwhile, take the slices of bread and toast them on one side only, giving them a circular shape, then spread the butter on the non-toasted side. Spread the buttered part of the bread with the mixture prepared previously, then sprinkle with a tablespoon of grated Parmesan cheese and bake at 200° for about 10 minutes, or wait for the cheese to melt. As soon as the bread is ready, garnish with thin slices of fresh tomato and serve immediately.

SHRIMP SANDWICH

for 4 people INGREDIENTS

- 4 sandwich

- 1/2 onion

- 1 jar of shrimps

- 4 cheese slices

- 1 knob of butter

- 1 tablespoon of mustard

PREPARATION

Drain the prawns. Take the sandwiches and cut them in half, then spread the butter and season with a slice of cheese. Then take an onion and chop it, add some mustard and add the prawns. Cover the sandwiches with parchment paper or parchment paper and let them rest for 20 minutes until served.

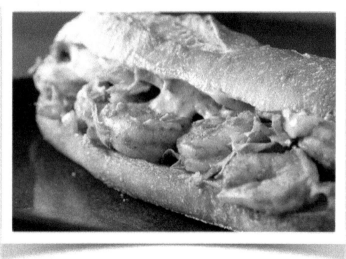

SALMON SANDWICH

for 4 people INGREDIENTS

- 4 sandwich

- 4 slices of smoked salmon

- 100 g of canned salmon

- Worcestershire sauce

- a little broth

- the juice of 1 lemon

- mayonnaise

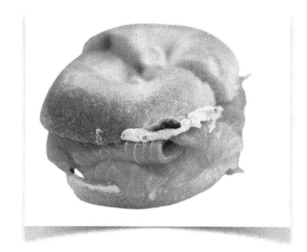

PREPARATION

Cut the sandwiches in half and empty the top of the crumb. Take a bowl and put the Worcestershire sauce, salmon, a little cold broth and mix everything with a blender. At the end transfer the mixture to a bowl and mix well, add the mayonnaise. After preparing the mixture, stuff the sandwiches and combine them with their upper part. To serve.

HERRING SANDWICH

for 4 people INGREDIENTS

- 4 sandwich

- 200 g of butter

- 2 tablespoons of mustard

- 4 herring fillets

PREPARATION

Melt the butter and mix it with the mustard. Immediately after, peel the herring fillets and grill them to the right point, but do not let them dry. Then take the sandwiches, sprinkle them with mustard butter, and put the herring fillets on top. Close the sandwiches and serve.

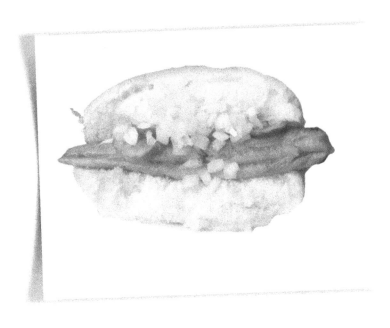

SARDINES AND BACON SANDWICH

for 4 people INGREDIENTS

- 4 sandwiches

- 1 can of sardines

- 4 slices of smoked bacon

- 2 fresh cheese

- 1 tablespoon of capers

- 1 teaspoon of paprika

- the juice of 1 lemon

- 1 knob of butter

PREPARATION

Take a bowl, drain the sardines and add the cheeses working them with a wooden ladle, now add the chopped capers, paprika and lemon juice and mix all the ingredients well. Take the sandwiches and cut them in half, then spread the butter and fill the sandwiches with the mixture.

Take a pan and fry the bacon, then place it in the center of the sandwich. Finally close the sandwiches with the top and wrap them with aluminum foil until served.

SANDWICH WITH BOILED FISH

for 4 people INGREDIENTS

- 8 slices of sandwich bread

- 100 g of boiled fish pulp

- 2 desalted anchovy fillets

- 50 g of butter 1 tablespoon of oil

- the juice of 1/2 lemon

- 1 teaspoon of capers - pepper

PREPARATION

Remove the bones from the anchovy fillets and season with oil, pepper, and lemon juice, then chop everything until the mixture becomes creamy. Finally, chop the capers and sprinkle them on the fish pulp. Now spread the ready mixture on the slices of bread and cover it with the top and serve.

TUNA AND MAYONNAISE SANDWICH

for 4 people INGREDIENTS

- 8 sandwiches

- 120 g of tuna in oil

- 5 tablespoons of mayonnaise sauce

- 1/2 tablespoon of chopped parsley

PREPARATION

After draining the oil from the tuna, chop it. Now cut the sandwiches in half and spread the lower part with mayonnaise, immediately afterwards lay the tuna and add the chopped parsley. Finally, cover the sandwiches with the other half and leave them to flavor for about an hour. Serve.

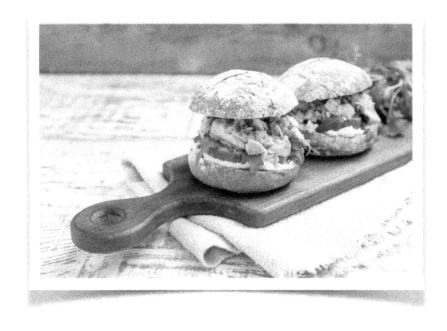

SEA TASTE SANDWICH

for 4 people INGREDIENTS

- 8 sandwiches

- 400 g of fresh or frozen mussels

- 2 cloves of garlic - oil

- 1 sprig of parsley

- 200 g of chopped tomato pulp - salt, pepper

PREPARATION

After washing the fresh mussels, put them to cook in a pan with oil and minced garlic, stir occasionally during the cooking period. As soon as the broth starts to boil, add the parsley, salt and finally plenty of pepper and cook for about 10/15 minutes, depending on the flame.

In the meantime that the mussels are cooking, cut the sandwiches in half and remove the top, now take the tomato pulp and drain it, add oil, salt and distribute it on the sandwiches. Pepper and bake in the oven at 200 ° for about 7/8 minutes. Remove the sandwiches from the oven and add the sauce with the mussels, refit the sandwich and serve hot.

CAVIAR AND VODKA SANDWICH

for 4 people INGREDIENTS

- 4 sandwiches

- 100 g of caviar

- 100 g of butter

- 15 anchovy fillets

- 1 tablespoon of vodka

PREPARATION

Take the anchovy fillets, and after removing the bones, put them in a mortar and mash them. Then prepare the butter making it creamier and add the vodka and anchovies.

Finally, cut the sandwiches and spread them on the mixture prepared with the anchovies, and add a spoonful of caviar.

Gently crush the sandwiches and serve.

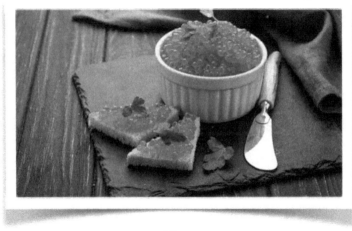

SAN JUAN SANDWICH

for 4 people INGREDIENTS

- 4 round rolls (sandwiches) - 1 box of crabmeat

- 40 g of chopped celery

- 40 g of chopped cucumbers

- 1 boiled egg

- 1 finely chopped shallot

- 60 g mayonnaise

- 1 large tomato

- 4 slices of savory cheese - paprika, chopped parsley

PREPARATION

Take the sandwiches, cut them in half and toast them. Then drain the crab meat and clean it of cartilage residues. Cut the sandwiches into slices and toast them in the oven. Meanwhile, mix the crab meat with the cucumber, egg, celery, mayonnaise and shallot. Now cut the tomato into slices and arrange them in the four halves of the sandwich, then take the crab meat with a spoon and distribute it on the tomato slice, add a slice of cheese and a pinch of paprika.

Finally, grill half of the sandwich with the mixture. When cooked, recompose the sandwich with the other half and serve..

SARDINES AND GROVIERA (CHEES) SANDWICH

for 4 people INGREDIENTS

- 4 sandwiches

- 150 g of canned sardines in oil

- 4 rosettes

- 75 g grated gruyere

- 120 ml white wine vinegar

- 1 small onion, thinly sliced

PREPARATION

Take three ice cubes and put them in a bowl with the onions and add the vinegar, then leave to act for about 15 minutes. Drain the sardines, but be careful to keep the oil. Now remove the crumb at the top of the sandwich. Then take the sandwich, fill it with sardines and add a drizzle of oil. Bring the oven to 200° and bake the sandwiches, but first add a slice of cheese and let it cook for 5 minutes until the cheese has melted. Finally, as soon as the sandwiches are ready, place them on a well heated plate, add the onion rings on top and serve immediately.

SEAFOOD SANDWICH

for 4 people INGREDIENTS

- 4 milk sandwiches
- 8 lettuce leaves
- 2 thinly sliced spring onions
- 3 finely chopped garlic cloves
- 2 teaspoons of curry
- 3 tablespoons of lemon juice
- 2 and 1/2 tablespoons of extra virgin olive oil
- 2 tablespoons of sauce Aurora
- fresh thyme
- 150 g of shrimp
- 150 g of cuttlefish
- 800 g of mussels
- 50 ml of brandy salt and pepper

PREPARATION

Wash the mussels and cuttlefish leaving them immersed in salted water for half an hour. Shell the prawns. After letting the mussels rest in plenty of salted water, put them in a pan with lemon juice and oil, and brown them until their shells open. Then fry the onions with a little garlic and brown the shrimp and cuttlefish, then add the brandy and cook for another 5/6 minutes. Then take the mussels with the sauce you prepared earlier and add the thyme leaves and curry, continue to cook for another 5 minutes.

Finally, cut the salad into small pieces and pour the remaining lemon juice and oil over it, so as to mix the mixture.

Now cut the sandwiches in half and fill them. Serve immediately.

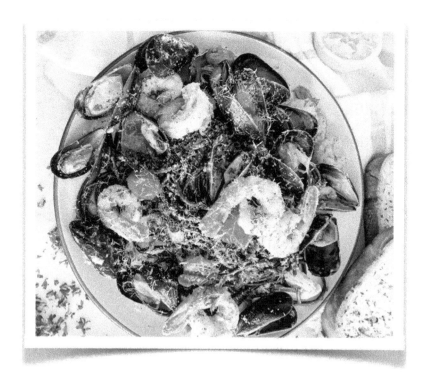

CAVIAR BUTTER SANDWICH

for 4 people INGREDIENTS

- 1 sandwich sliced loaf pan 1/2

- 100 g. butter

- 100 g of caviar

- lemon slices

PREPARATION

Cut the sandwiches and remove the crust, then divide them into triangles. Pass the butter with the caviar in a pan to obtain a tasty homogeneous cream. Then spread the cream on the slices of bread and season to your liking.

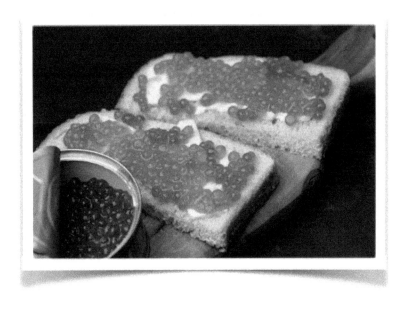

CAVIAR SANDWICH

for 4 people INGREDIENTS

- 4 slices of bread in a box

- 200 g of butter

- 1 hard-boiled egg

- 1/2 grated onion

- 1 jar of caviar

PREPARATION

Take the sandwiches and divide them in half and spread the butter on the bottom of the sandwich. Take the hard-boiled egg and put it together with the grated onion on the sandwich, then add a spoonful of caviar. served.

SMOKED SALMON SANDWICH

for 4 people INGREDIENTS

- 8 slices of bread

- 80 g smoked salmon cut into slices

- 40 g of butter

- lemon juice

- 4 lemon slices, peeled and cut into triangles

- freshly ground pepper

PREPARATION

Take the sandwiches and remove the crust, then mix the butter and a little lemon juice. Now spread the mixture obtained previously and spread it on the four slices of bread, then cover the bread with the slices of salmon and add a little lemon pulp and spices to your liking. Serve

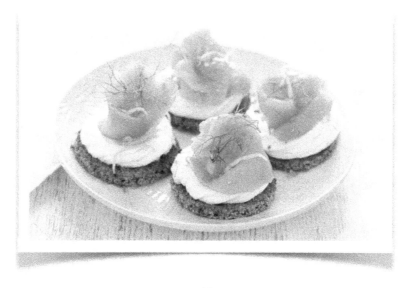

LOBSTER SANDWICH

for 4 people INGREDIENTS

- 4 sandwiches

- 50 g of butter

- 50 g of grated cheese

- 2 hard-boiled egg yolks

- 1 tablespoon of mustard

- pieces of boiled lobster

- salt

PREPARATION

Take a bowl and melt the cheese, butter and crumbled egg yolks in it until you get a creamy and homogeneous compost.

Then add the mustard, adjusting the mixture with a pinch of salt and mix slowly. In the meantime, open the sandwiches in two parts and spread the cream you just prepared, add pieces of boiled lobster. Serve.

ANCHOVIES SANDWICH

for 4 people INGREDIENTS

- 4 sandwiches

- 50 g of butter

- 100 g anchovies fillets

- pepper

- capers

PREPARATION

Take a mortar and prepare the anchovies by working them with 80 grams of anchovies and butter, also add the pepper. In the meantime, remove the crumbs from the sandwiches and spread the anchovies prepared with a mortar on top. Arrange the sandwiches on a serving dish and add a rolled fillet to each sandwich, finally add the capers. Serve.

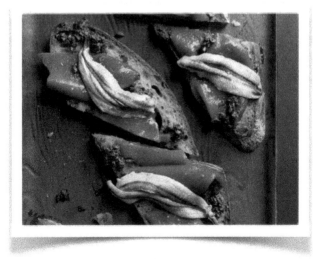

STURGEON SANDWICH

for 4 people INGREDIENTS

- 8 very thin slices of rye bread

- 4 slices of smoked sturgeon

- 4 teaspoons of caviar or lumpfish egg

- butter

- fresh chive strands

- lemon

- pepper

PREPARATION

Take a plate with the highest edges, now take the sturgeon slices and sprinkle them with lemon juice, season with freshly ground pepper and leave to flavor for about 50 minutes. After draining the sturgeon, take the slices of bread and arrange it on a serving dish and arrange the sturgeon on each slice, lightly butter and add a spoonful of caviar and chives. Close the four slices of bread with the remaining slices. Serve.

DANISH SANDWICH

for 6 people INGREDIENTS

- 6 slices of sandwich bread
- 250 g cooked lobster, crab or shrimp pulp
- 1 small jar of black or red caviar
- 3 hard-boiled eggs
- 6 lettuce leaves
- 1 tablespoon of mayonnaise
- a pinch of mustard powder
- butter to garnish: tomato wedges - parsley sprigs - lemon wedges

PREPARATION

After having properly toasted the slices of bread, spread the butter on one side. Add a lettuce leaf and with a spoon pour the shellfish pulp on the slices and add a spoonful of black caviar. Meanwhile, cut the eggs into two parts and remove the yolk. Take a bowl and put the mustard with the mayonnaise and add the previously removed yolk and mix until you get a creamy mixture. Now fill the half eggs with the mixture obtained. Finally, put the half egg in the center of the caviar with the addition of parsley. Arrange the sandwiches on a serving dish and garnish with pieces of tomato, lemon, and parsley sprigs.

SARDINES SANDWICH

for 4 people INGREDIENTS

- 8 slices of bread100 g of butter

- 1 tablespoon of anchovy paste

- 100 g of tuna in oil

- 1 tin of sardines without bones

- parsley, chopped onion

PREPARATION

Take the tuna and crumble it, then add the butter with the anchovy paste, the sardines, the parsley. finely chopped onion and mix until a consistent mixture is obtained. Finally spread the slices of bread with the creamy mixture and cover them with the other slices. Serve on a serving plate.

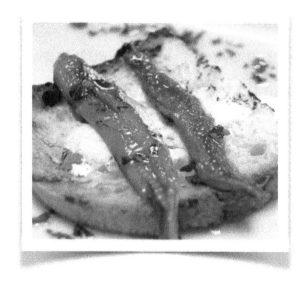

OYSTER SANDWICH

for 4 people INGREDIENTS

- 8 very thin slices of whole grain bread
- 8 large oysters
- 2 tablespoons of mustard
- 1 tablespoon of ketchup sauce
- 40 g of butter
- lemon
- parsley
- salt and pepper

PREPARATION

Open the oysters and place them in a container, keeping the liquid. Take a bowl and work the butter together with a sprinkling of ground pepper, a pinch of salt and finally add a few drops of oyster liquid, then mix until you get a creamy mixture. Prepare the slices of bread and spread the butter on them, take the oysters with a spoon and put them on all four slices of bread, add the parsley and a squeeze of lemon. Finally, make a mixture of butter, hot sauce, and mustard to garnish the sandwich. Put the sandwiches obtained in the fridge until you serve them.

TUNA AND ROASTED PEPPER SANDWICH

for 6 people INGREDIENTS

- 1 large flat bread with thyme or rosemary or

- 6 rolls of Arab bread

- 200 g tuna in oil

- 3 large peeled roasted red peppers

- 2 tablespoons of lemon juice

- 1 teaspoon of finely chopped fresh thyme

- 50 ml plus 2 tablespoons of extra virgin olive oil

- 120 g of parsley leaves1 thinly sliced red onion

- 2 tablespoons of capers salt and pepper

PREPARATION

Drain the tuna and put it in a bowl with a little lemon juice, onion, thyme, salt and pepper as required. Take another bowl and put the remaining tuna with oil, parsley and always season with salt and pepper.

At this point, cut the focaccia in half and fill it with the slices of roasted pepper and the mixture obtained previously. Finally, cover the focaccia with the other half and put it in the fridge covered with plastic wrap for about 50 minutes. Before serving, cut it into wedges.

MUSHROOM CROUTONS

for 4 people INGREDIENTS

- 1/2 kg of thinly sliced cultivated mushrooms

- 4 slices of homemade bread

- 3 and a half tablespoons of butter

- 2 tablespoons of flour 3.5 dl of milk

- 1.5 dl of dry white wine

- 4 teaspoons of finely chopped onion

- 1 tablespoon of soy sauce

- 2 tablespoons of brandy grated parmesan

- salt

- pepper

PREPARATION

Take a medium-sized pan and melt a tablespoon of butter, add the flour and cook over low heat for about 4 minutes. Meanwhile, stir slowly and add the milk and the wine, mix it slowly with a ladle and wait for the sauce to thicken, season with salt and pepper, then cook for another 14 minutes.

Take another pan and sprinkle it with butter, let it heat up, add the mushrooms and let them brown for about 3 minutes.

Now take the heated brandy, set the pan on fire until the flames have gone out.

Place the four slices of bread in the bowls and pour the mushrooms over them, then sprinkle with the sauce and grated Parmesan.

Cook everything at 200° for about 10 minutes waiting for the cheese to melt and turn slightly golden. Serve.

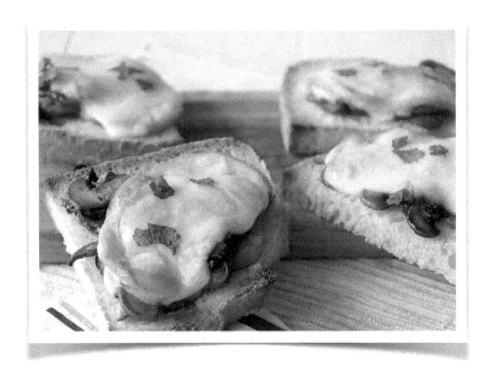

BLACK OLIVE CROUTONS

for 10 people INGREDIENTS

- 10 round rolls

- 150 g of pitted and chopped black olives

- 100 g of mayonnaise

- 2 tablespoons of finely chopped onion

- 150 g of grated Gruyere cheese

- 1/2 teaspoon of curry powder

PREPARATION

Take the sandwiches, cut them in two and toast them. Then take a bowl where you will go to work the mayonnaise, olives, onion, curry and cheese. Take the sandwiches and divide the mixture obtained previously and sprinkle it on the toasted sandwiches, then place them on the grill and cook for about 4 minutes. finally take a serving dish and arrange the sandwiches before serving.

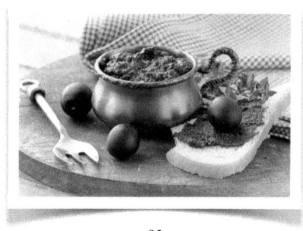

TOMATO SANDWICH

for 4 people INGREDIENTS

- 4 slices of homemade bread

- 4 thick slices of ripe tomatoes

- 4 thin slices of fontina

- butter

- mayonnaise

- Dijon mustard

PREPARATION

After toasting the slices of bread on one side only, spread the untoasted side with the butter, mustard and mayonnaise. Finally add a slice of cheese and a slice of tomato. Then grill it until the cheese has melted or turns slightly golden. Then serve.

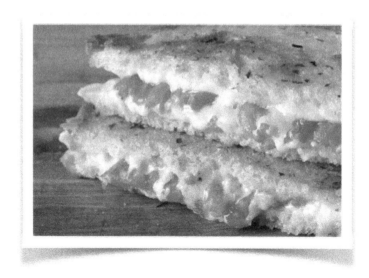

PAN BAGNAT NIZZA

for 4 people INGREDIENTS

- 4 large slices of stale Tuscan or Apulian homemade bread

- 4 ripe and firm tomatoes

- 2 tablespoons of vinegar

- 2 tablespoons of virgin olive oil - lettuce leaves - black olives

onion rings - fresh basil - salt and pepper

PREPARATION

Fill a glass of cold water, place the slices of bread on a large plate, wet them and let them rest for about 20 minutes until the water is absorbed by the slices of bread. After 20 minutes, remove the excess water, but be careful that the slices remain intact. Now take a serving dish and spread out the slices of bread, then put a lettuce leaf on top, the sliced tomato and season with oil, salt and vinegar. Before serving, garnish with black olives, onion, basil leaves and leave to rest for 15 minutes before serving.

CARRETERA SANDWICH

for 4 people INGREDIENTS

- 4 sandwiches

- fresh tomatoes

- garlic, chopped basil

- oil, salt, pepper

PREPARATION

Cut the sandwiches in half, then put them to toast for a few minutes. Meanwhile, chop the tomatoes and mix with oil, pepper, salt, basil and garlic, mix everything with a wooden spoon and season while still hot, remember to remove the garlic. Before closing the sandwich with the other half you can still add a drizzle of oil, salt and pepper to flavor the top of the sandwich. Arrange the sandwiches on a serving dish and serve immediately.

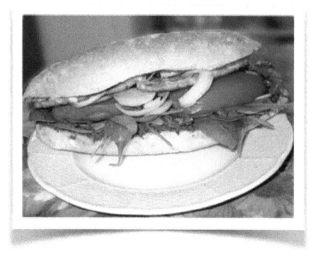

AGRO SANDWICH

for 4 people INGREDIENTS

- 4 slices of bread

- green salad

- 70 g of butter

- parsley

- the juice of 1 lemon, salt

PREPARATION

Take a cup of milk and add the lemon juice, parsley, butter and mix everything until you get a homogeneous mixture. Meanwhile, toast the slices of bread in the oven for 6/7 minutes, as soon as they come out of the oven spread a layer of butter and immediately add the mixture with the lemon, now garnish the slice of bread with the green salad and serve.

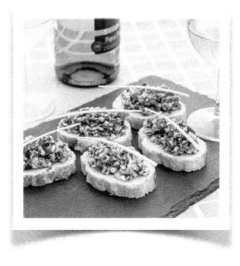

MIXED VEGETABLE SANDWICH

for 4 people INGREDIENTS

- 4 sandwiches

- 70 g of butter

- 2 carrots

- 2-3 courgettes

- 2 handfuls of peas

- 1 cup of broth

PREPARATION

Cut the sandwiches in two and remove the crumb. Put the vegetables in a pan and boil for a few minutes, as soon as the water starts to evaporate, put the butter in the pan and brown the vegetables. Spread the butter inside the sandwiches and add the browned vegetables. Now take a pan, dust it with butter and place the sandwiches on the bottom, pour the broth over it and sprinkle it on the sandwiches, now wait for them to become crispy. When the sandwiches are ready, place them on a serving dish and serve..

RUSSIAN SALAD SANDWICH

for 8 people INGREDIENTS

- 8 milk rolls

- 130 g Russian salad

- 2 tablespoons of mayonnaise

- 8 small lettuce leaves

PREPARATION

Wash the lettuce and dry it.

Take the sandwiches and split them in half, immediately spread the mayonnaise on both sides and put a lettuce leaf inside them, then take the Russian salad and put it in the middle. Finally, lightly press the sandwiches and serve.

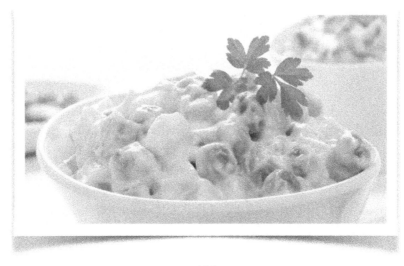

MEDITERRANEAN SANDWICH

for 6 people INGREDIENTS

- 1 narrow loaf or 1 baguette

- 400 g of coarsely chopped tomato pulp

- 100 g of thinly sliced shallot

- 50 g of green olives stuffed with pepper, chopped

- 50 g of pitted and chopped black olives

- 30 g of chopped parsley

- 1 teaspoon of chopped fresh thyme or 1 pinch of dried one

- 1 tablespoon of capers

- 1 tablespoon of chopped basil

- 2-3 tablespoons of olive oil - salt, pepper

PREPARATION

Remove the two ends from the loaf by cutting them with a knife and remove the crumb inside them, chop the remaining excess crumb with a food processor.

Take a large bowl and mix the tomato, black olives, capers, green olives, basil, thyme, parsley, shallot, and the crumb, now add the oil to soften the mixture, finally salt and pepper. just enough.

As soon as the mixture is ready, fill the loaf and wrap it in aluminum foil and put it in the fridge for at least seven hours or overnight. Before serving, take it out of the fridge at least an hour before, slice and distribute the sandwiches.

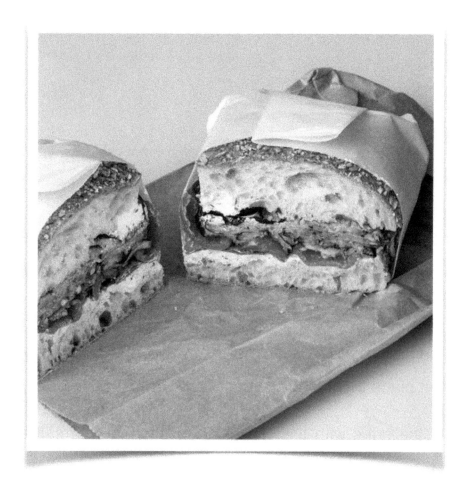

DELICIOUS SANDWICH

for 4 people INGREDIENTS

- 8 milk sandwiches - 4 eggs

- 150 g of champignons - 1 shallot

- 50 g of butter

- 3 tablespoons of cream

- 1 tablespoon of tomato sauce

- Tabasco

- salt

- pepper

PREPARATION

Cut the mushrooms and chop them, then take a pan and put 20 grams of butter in it, add the shallot and brown. While cooking, season with salt and pepper and cook for about 12 minutes, add a few drops of Tabasco and tomato.

In the meantime, cut the sandwiches in two and brush the inside with butter, then place them in the oven to lightly toast at 175 degrees.

Now beat the eggs with the cream, then season with salt and pepper, now add the mixture that you had previously prepared.

Finally, take the sandwiches out of the oven, take the mixture obtained and distribute it inside the sandwiches, close with the other half and serve.

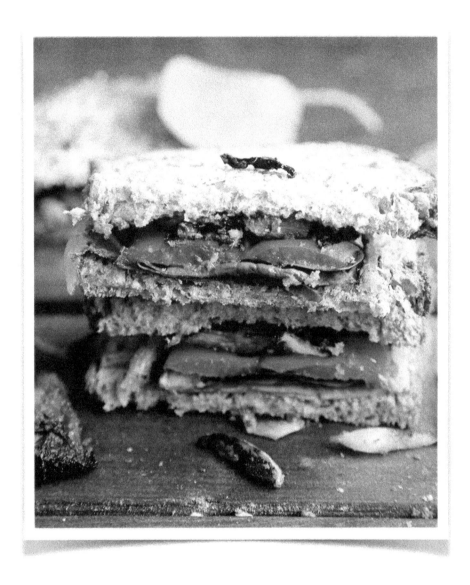

VEGETARIAN SANDWICH

for 8 people INGREDIENTS

- 8 milk rolls

- 2 hard boiled eggs

- 1 fennel

- 2 tomatoes

- 2 layers of green pepper in oil

- 2 sticks of celery

- 130 g of tuna in oil

- 8 anchovies stuffed with capers

- 8 olives stuffed with peppers

- 1 tablespoon of mayonnaise

- 1 pack of white yogurt

- 1 teaspoon of Worcestershire sauce

- chives

- salt and pepper

PREPARATION

Cut the sandwiches in half and remove the crumb. Now cut the pepper, the fennel and chop the tomato with the celery. Meanwhile, drain the tuna and mix all the ingredients in a bowl.

Fill the sandwiches with this topping. In another bowl pour the Worcestershire sauce, yogurt, and chives, mix everything, then season with salt and pepper.

Then garnish the top of the sandwiches with a wedge of hard-boiled egg, an olive, and capers.

Finally, put the sauce made with yogurt in a separate bowl and serve the sandwiches on a serving dish.

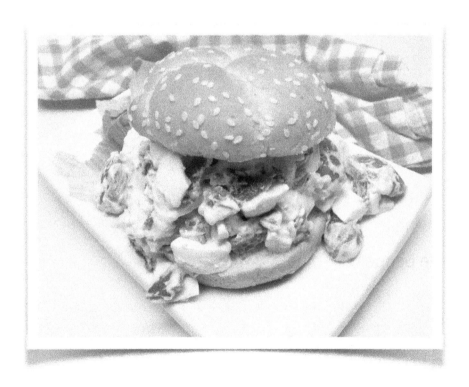

SANDWICH WITH MEATBALLS

for 4 people INGREDIENTS

- 4 "pita" sandwiches

- 200 g of naturally boiled chickpeas

- 4 pinches of coriander

- 4 pinches of cumin

- 2 cloves of garlic

- 8 lettuce leaves

- 3-4 ripe tomatoes

- 3 tablespoons of tahini (sesame seed paste)

- 1 tablespoon of sesame seeds

- parsley

- 1/2 teaspoon of paprika

- 1 red pepper

- 1 tablespoon of lemon juice

- flour

- oil for frying

- cayenne pepper

- salt

PREPARATION

Start with preparing the meatballs. Take a food processor and blend the chickpeas, place them in a bowl and toss with the cumin, finely chopped garlic, coriander and salt and cayenne pepper. As soon as the mixture is ready, let it rest for 30 minutes, prepare the meatballs, mash them and cover with flour.

Now prepare the sauce with the tahini, parsley, lemon juice, a finely chopped clove of garlic, paprika, a pinch of salt and mix. At this point, fry the meatballs in oil and drain them in absorbent paper. Remove the breadcrumbs and stuff them with a lettuce leaf, sliced pepper and tomato. Now season the meatballs with the tahini sauce and place them in the center of the sandwich. Serve.

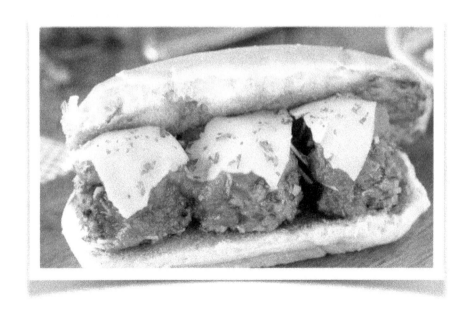

ENGLISH SANDWICH

for 6 people INGREDIENTS - 2 cucumbers

- 1 teaspoon of white vinegar

- 1/2 teaspoon of salt

- 6 very thin slices of dark bread

- butter

PREPARATION

Cut 40 discs of very thin cucumbers, mix them with the vinegar and let them rest for 30 minutes so that they lose their water.

With a mold, cut four discs from the slices of bread and spread a layer of butter on them. Season the bread with the cucumber discs and cover them with the other half. As soon as they are ready, put them in the fridge to rest for 30 minutes covered with a damp cloth. Finally arrange them on a serving dish and serve.

MUSHROOMS SANDWICH

for 4 people INGREDIENTS

- 16 medium sized porcini mushrooms

- 200 g of roasted meat leftovers

- 90 g of lard

- 30 g of butter

- 1 stale milk sandwich

- 3 eggs

- 50 g of grated Parmesan cheese

- milk

- breadcrumbs

- flour

- parsley

- salt

PREPARATION

Clean the mushrooms, remove the stems and chop them in half, because we will use them for two different dishes. Brown the mushrooms in a pan with 30 grams of lard and butter for about 12 minutes. Meanwhile pass the meat with the food processor. Take a bowl and pour in the breadcrumbs, milk, mushroom stem, minced meat, chopped parsley, an egg and grated Parmesan. At this point season the mushroom-shaped chapels with a pinch of salt and spread the previously worked mixture on them, then pass them in the flour, then in the beaten eggs and again in the breadcrumbs.

Put them to cook in the lard, turning them often and browning them until they become golden and crunchy. As soon as the mushrooms are cooked, let them drain for a few minutes in the absorbent paper.

Now put them on a serving dish and serve hot.

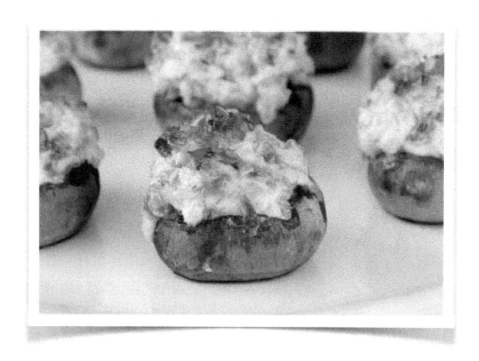

EGGPLANT SANDWICH

for 4 people INGREDIENTS

- 3 aubergines

- tomato sauce made with 1/2 kg of tomatoes

- basil, garlic, onion, oil

- 150 g of thin slices of cheese

- 2 eggs - flour breadcrumbs

- oil for frying - salt

PREPARATION

Slice the aubergines and sprinkle them with salt so that they lose excess water. Now take a slice of aubergine and spread the tomato sauce over it and close it with another slice of aubergine, pass the sandwich in the flour, then in the egg, and then in the breadcrumbs. Finally, prepare the rest of the aubergines in the same way and fry them in a pan with hot oil until cooked. As soon as the eggplant sandwiches are ready, drain them with absorbent paper. To serve.

POTATO SANDWICH

for 4 people INGREDIENTS

- 1 kg of potatoes

- 100 g of butter - 200 g of sliced cooked ham

- 100 g of grated Emmental

- other cheese cut into thin slices - 2 eggs, flour, salt

PREPARATION

After having peeled the potatoes, boil them in salted water and as soon as they are ready, mash them until a homogeneous puree is obtained. Now take a pastry board and flour it, put the mashed potatoes and add a knob of butter, the eggs and mix well, finally level the puree mixture to a thickness of one centimeter, flour it and let it rest for about 30 minutes. When the mashed potatoes have cooled and are more compact, cut them into rectangles.

Then take a pan and sprinkle it with butter, as soon as it is hot put the crushed balls in it until the pan is full, then put on each rectangle half a slice of ham and the cheese cut into rectangles of the same shape as the puree, to finish cover all the rectangles of the pan well.

Now take a saucepan from the oven and butter it, then put in the loaves that were in the pan. Cover with grated Emmental and butter flakes and bake in the oven at 180° for about half an hour. Finally, arrange the sandwiches on a serving dish and serve.

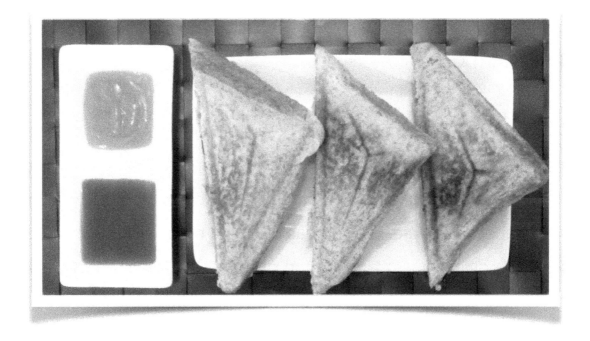

TOMATO SANDWICH

for 3 or 6 people INGREDIENTS

- large tomatoes

- 180 g of soft white cheese like Philadelphia

- 2 tablespoons of cream

- 1 clove of garlic

- 1 egg - 120 g of breadcrumbs

- 2 tablespoons of butter - salt

PREPARATION

Cut 12 slices of tomato about 1 centimeter thick, spread them on absorbent paper and let them dry for five minutes. Take a bowl and put the cheese, chopped garlic, cream and mix well until you get a homogeneous mixture. Now spread 6 tomato slices with the mixture and place the other tomato slice on top of each slice. Beat an egg and dip the tomato sandwiches in it, dip them in the breadcrumbs, do it with the rest of the tomato sandwiches. Take a pan and butter it, dip the tomato sandwiches and cook for about 3 minutes until golden brown. Finally, place them on a serving dish and put a pinch of salt in them. Now serve.

VEGETABLE SANDWICH

for 6 people INGREDIENTS

- 6 slices of bread

- 80 g of chopped cabbage

- 80 g of chopped carrots

- 50 g of chopped green pepper

- 50 g of chopped celery

- 50 g of chopped radishes

- 100 g of chopped sweet onion

- 400 g of grated Parmesan cheese

- 1/2 cup of beer

- butter

- White pepper

- cayenne

- pepper

- salt

PREPARATION

Take a bowl and put the carrots, pepper, celery, radishes, cabbage and onion in it, season with salt and mix well. Meanwhile, toast the slices of bread and, as soon as they are ready, spread the butter on them and place the vegetable mixture on them.

Put the tomato sauce and cheese in a separate pan, cook until you get a thick and homogeneous sauce. Now take a saucepan and sprinkle it with butter, take the slices of bread and put them in the casserole, put the cheese sauce on top and simmer them for 3 minutes until the cheese has melted on the slices. Serve.

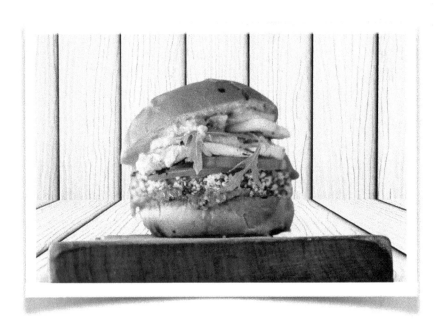

MIXED MEAT SANDWICH

for 4 people INGREDIENTS

- 12 slices of sandwich bread

- 200 g of meat, chicken or turkey cooked thinly sliced

- 3 firm and ripe tomatoes sliced and without seeds

- 4 slices of cooked ham

- butter 1/2 liter of mayonnaise

- 1/2 teaspoon of Dijon mustard

- lettuce leaves

- 8 strips of crispy fried bacon

- 4 large black or green olives

PREPARATION

Toast 8 slices of bread, take four and use them as a base for sandwiches. Mix the mayonnaise with the mustard. On the base put a slice of chicken with mayonnaise, a little lettuce, a slice of tomato and a strip of bacon, now overlap a slice of buttered bread with a little mayonnaise and add another slice of cooked ham, a slice of tomato, one of bacon; finally cover everything with another toasted slice. Do the same with the other slices of bread. Decorate the sandwiches with a toothpick and an olive.

BRAZILIAN SANDWICH

for 4 people INGREDIENTS

- 3 bananas

- 150 g of very lean cooked ham

- 2 stalks of very white celery

- 8 slices of sandwich bread

- 1 onion - 1 tablespoon of Dijon mustard

- 2-3 tablespoons of butter

PREPARATION

Cut the ham into small pieces, chop the celery and onion, cut the banana and mix everything in the food processor to obtain a homogeneous puree. Now work the butter with the mustard and spread it on the four slices of bread. Then take the mixture obtained from the banana and distribute it over the sandwich, now recompose the sandwich with the other slices of bread and serve it.

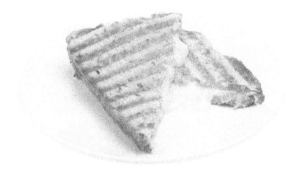

AVOCADO SANDWICH

for 4 people INGREDIENTS

- 2 ripe avocados

- 4 "pita" bread rolls

- 100 g finely chopped shallot

- 2 peeled tomatoes with seeds removed and coarsely chopped

- 3 tablespoons of lemon juice

- 1 tablespoon of coriander

- 1/2 teaspoon of chili powder

- Tabasco lettuce leaves

- salt, pepper

PREPARATION

Peel the avocados, remove the stone and mash the pulp; add the shallot, lemon juice, chili, tomato, coriander, tabasco, salt, and pepper as required. Finally, mix well until you get a thick cream. Now cut the sandwiches in half, put a lettuce leaf in the center, and spread the previously prepared mixture over it. Serve immediately.

EGG AND ANCHOVIES SANDWICH

for 4 people INGREDIENTS

- 3 hard-boiled eggs

- 8 thin slices of very fresh sandwich bread

- 4 anchovy fillets

- 60 g of butter

- 1/2 teaspoon of finely chopped onion

- 1 tablespoon of mayonnaise

- 1 teaspoon of Dijon mustard

- salt and pepper

- sprigs of cress for garnish

PREPARATION

Take a bowl and put the chopped hard-boiled eggs, the chopped anchovy fillets, the butter, the onion, the mayonnaise, the mustard, a pinch of salt and pepper, now mix well until the mixture is well blended. As soon as the mixture is ready, divide the sandwiches in half and butter the inside of the upper part of the sandwiches, then spread the previously prepared mixture and close them with the other half of the sandwiches, do it with all the other sandwiches. Arrange them on a serving plate and cut them into a triangular shape. To serve.

EGG AND BASIL SANDWICH

- for 4 people INGREDIENTS

- 8 slices of wholemeal bread

- 3 hard-boiled eggs

- 3 tablespoons of butter

- 1 tablespoon of finely chopped basil

- 4 black olives a few fillets of red pepper in oil

PREPARATION

Toast the slices of bread, in the meantime work the butter with the basil, until a homogeneous cream is obtained. As soon as the cream is ready, divide the sandwiches in half and spread it on both slices, at this point add the pitted black olives, and the pepper fillets in oil. Finally close the sandwiches with their upper part. To serve.

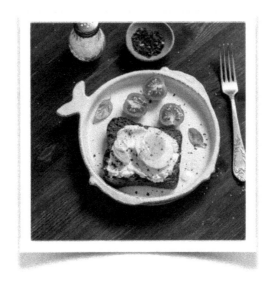

EGG AND CHIVE SANDWICH

for 4 people INGREDIENTS

- 4 hard-boiled eggs

- 3 tablespoons of chopped fresh chives

- 2 tablespoons of mayonnaise

- 6 tablespoons of butter

- 1 and 1/2 teaspoons of anchovy paste

- 8 thin slices of sliced bread - salt, pepper,

- sprigs of parsley for garnish

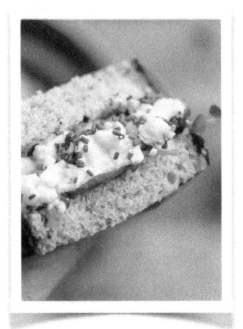

PREPARATION

Spread the butter with the anchovy and pepper paste just enough. With a knife chop the hard-boiled eggs and put them in a bowl together with mayonnaise, chives, salt and pepper; mix well until you get a homogeneous mixture.

Divide the sandwiches in half and spread the egg mixture on the four slices and cover with the other slices with the buttered side facing down. If you want you can also remove the crust from the bread, cut the sandwiches into triangles and arrange them on a serving dish. Before serving the sandwiches you can garnish with parsley sprigs and serve.

AMERICAN HAZELNUT SANDWICH

for 4 people INGREDIENTS

- 8 slices of sandwich bread

- 12 freshly toasted American peanuts

- 150 g of Roman ricotta

- 1 pinch of chili powder, salt

PREPARATION

After finely chopping the peanuts in the food processor, sift the ricotta and place it in a bowl. Add the peanuts, the pulverized chilli, a pinch of salt to the ricotta and mix the mixture well. Put the mixture in the fridge for at least 30 minutes and wait for it to thicken. Finally, take the four slices of bread and divide the mixture on them, reassemble the sandwiches and arrange them on a plate, cut them in half forming triangles and serve.

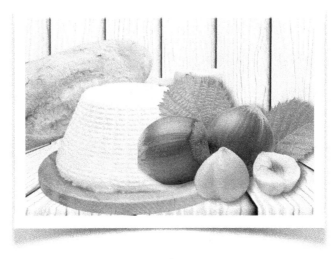

EGG SALAD SANDWICH WITH CURRY

for 4 people INGREDIENTS

- 5 boiled eggs

- 8 slices of wholemeal bread

- 2 tablespoons of butter

- 1 teaspoon of curry powder

- 50 g of mayonnaise

1 teaspoon of lemon juice

1 teaspoon of Dijon mustard

salt, pepper

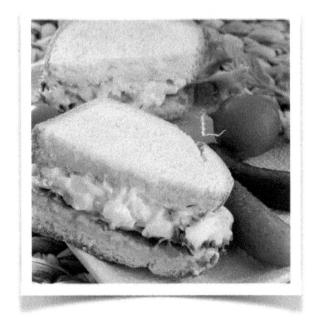

PREPARATION

Melt the butter in a saucepan, add the curry and cook for about a minute, stirring constantly. Let cool and add the mayonnaise, chopped eggs, lemon juice, mustard and season with a pinch of salt. Mix the mixture until smooth and spread it on the four slices of bread, close them with the other four slices and serve.

TASTY EGG SANDWICH

for 4 people INGREDIENTS

- 4 finely chopped hard-boiled eggs

- 8 slices of sandwich bread butter

- 1 teaspoon of mustard

- 1/2 teaspoon of onion powder Worcestershire sauce

- 1 tablespoon of chopped parsley

- 2 tablespoons of chopped pickled red peppers

- 2 teaspoons of vinegar

- 50 g of mayonnaise

- salt

- pepper

PREPARATION

Spread the slices of bread with butter. Take a bowl and mix the mustard, eggs, onion powder, a splash of Worcestershire sauce, pepperoni, parsley, vinegar, and mayonnaise; add salt and pepper. Divide the mixture over the four slices of bread and cover with the other slices. Take a serving dish and divide the sandwiches into triangles.